TABLE OF CONTENTS

THE M.E.L.T. STORY

Welcome to the m.e.l.t. family! I wrote this book because I want to help you realize how much you are actually capable of and to equip you with the tools you need to get (and keep) the body you want in less time.

What is m.e.l.t.? It's an acronym for *more energy, less time.*

More energy: You burn more energy (calories) from these workouts, have more energy throughout the day to be more productive and sleep better at night.

Less time: You get better results in less time through our 30 minute workouts.

At m.e.l.t. we transform our mind and body through "serious fun" sessions and small steps forward each day. Just commit to show up and give one percent more. At m.e.l.t., you'll love the positive energy, you'll find that the 30-minute workouts fly by, and you'll learn that living a healthy life style is not as hard as you thought.

Our credo is:

"We live one rep at a time. We become stronger with every movement and leaner than yesterday.

We are 20 times more capable because we believe in progress, not perfection.

We give to those less fortunate and support each other.

M.e.l.t. is a fitness community where you matter and belong.

Sweat. Smile. Live who you were meant to be. "

How it All Began

This story all started with a book no one has ever read: *How to Look Better Naked*, which Joe Carabase wrote while he was in college. At the time, Joe had trained for a couple years in various locations—on the University of Massachusetts Campus, in several Gold's Gyms throughout New England, and in a health club in Brisbane, Australia. Through his experience working with a diverse range of people—college kids, professors, business professionals, the elderly, and people with severe health issues, he realized that the training principles from one population to the other are not that different—it's just a matter of modifying accordingly.

Joe also began to realize that if the program is designed properly, 60-minute workouts are unnecessary. He gradually discovered how to deliver better results in less time. So, he figured, why not create a book for everyone to read to look better naked?

This was the moment the seed for m.e.l.t. was planted; he just didn't know its potential. Without researching how to publish or seeking professional advice, he wrote that book.

Joe quickly realized he had no idea what to do with his book. For some reason, big-time publishers were not knocking on his door! It became clear that he needed to go in a different direction. With the help of his uncle's web background and a 16-year-old from India whom Joe kept up late and woke up early to communicate with due to the time difference, he created the website www.carabasetraining.com.

During the second semester of Joe's senior year in college, he landed an internship at Gold's Gym in Amherst, Massachusetts, where he provided personal training while working on his website. Joe dreaded the 30-minute drive to Longmeadow (where he worked) and all he could think about when he was there was his website.

He knew there was something bigger for him out there, an opportunity to really make an impact and help a lot of people. Anxious, scared, but most of all inspired, Joe quit the internship, declined their full-time offer, and decided to start a training business upon graduating.

So with no money, no business plan, no clients and a few pairs of rusty old weights, Joe started his onsite training business out of his trunk.

For the next year, Joe traveled anywhere, trained anyone, and did anything he could to gain experience. His business operated under "Carabase Training," "Fit Body Bootcamp," "Fat Burning Bootcamp," and "The Fit Tribe." Joe had in-home clients in Stonington and Wallingford, Connecticut, a boot camp with one to five people at 20 Church Street in Hartford, and a boot camp with one to six people in South Windsor at varying locations. Some days Joe would be training five people, while on other days he trained one. And some days he trained no one, which was a feeling he will never forget.

During his first year in business, someone advised Joe to apply for a job as a Personal Training Instructor at Branford Hall Career Institute.

He started teaching part-time and shortly got promoted to direct the department, while trying to grow an onsite personal training business. Branford Hall was a great experience for Joe. It gave him HUGE respect for what teachers do day in and day out, year after year. He learned a lot about communicating a message, instructing people double (and even triple) his own age, and personal development. But the three best parts of that job ended up being the first three employees (who were students) at m.e.l.t, all of whom are still here changing people's lives daily: Nicole DiMauro, Aaron Granahan, and Sue Adams.

After a year and a half at Branford Hall, Joe hit a crossroad. He felt there was no more room for personal or professional growth, and he knew something had to change for his business or else it wouldn't survive. Joe attended a seminar in Kentucky and heard a quote that changed his life. Pat Rigsby, one of Joe's mentors, said, "You don't know your limits. Whatever limits you see are self-imposed. You can't fail if you learn from the situation." Something clicked. In that moment he decided to open his first location in South Windsor. The next week Joe signed a lease to start in two months.

Joe had a planned vacation to cruise the Caribbean right after signing the lease. On the boat, he was jotting down ideas for what he wanted the company to be about and what it was going to be called. After about an hour of writing, "m.e.l.t. more energy, less time" inspiration struck Joe. The phrase *more energy, less time* – **m.e.l.t.** – embodied his training philosophy and sounded pretty damn cool. Fast forward to today.

The original m.e.l.t. location in South Windsor opened in 2010. It later moved to a location three-and-a-half times the original size, and has some exciting renovations and future expansions planned. M.e.l.t. Glastonbury opened its doors in a tiny, long space in Spring 2011 and is now in a space 5 times the original size.

The Simsbury location opened in April 2014 and is growing by leaps and bounds every day! m.e.l.t. broke into the mobile market with its "m.e.l.t.30" FREE app launched in May 2013. The newest venture is the m.e.l.t.30 At Home Fat Loss &

Strength DVD, which includes nine m.e.l.t.-style, follow-along workouts: Upper & Lower Body Cardio Strengthening, Fat Burning Bootcamp (2x), Core & Cardio (2x), The "Push" & "Pull" Sculpt Series and m.e.l.t.ed Yoga. The DVD launched locally August 12, 2013, and became available online in early Fall 2014.

THE FOUR PARTS OF M.E.L.T.

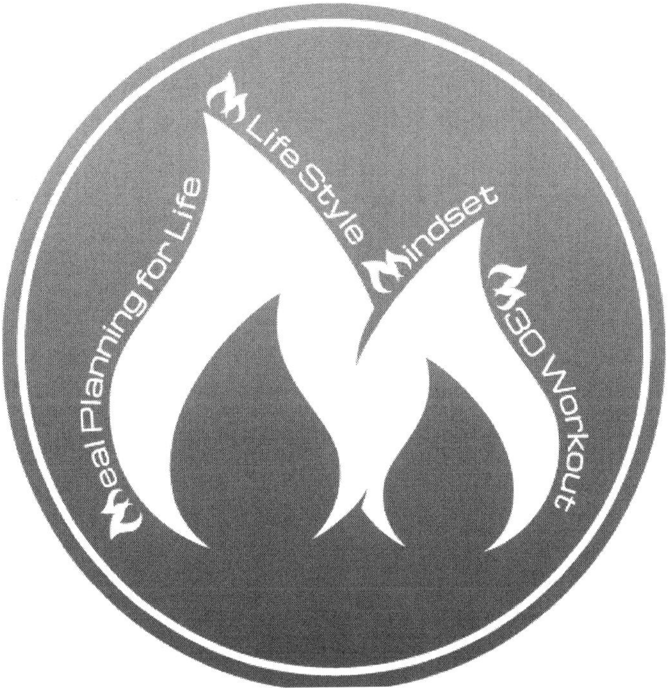

"You can fail at what you don't want and don't do so you might as well go for what you want"

— Jim Carrey's Dad

Have you ever signed up for a 1-year gym membership and only worked out one or two times? Have you ever bought an exercise DVD and watched it from the couch—and that's the last time you ever pressed Play? Have you ever jumped on the latest fitness craze—and maybe even saw some results for a while—but got incredibly bored and couldn't keep your interest going? And now you're feeling like a failure because you're always trying but never succeeding?

Well, I'm here to tell you it's NOT your fault.

Most gyms and exercise DVDs provide nothing but a generic workout. Some may give you "nutrition guidelines" that really end up being highly restrictive, unsustainable diets.

Trying to address your health with only repetitive workouts and a strict diet is like trying to sit on a chair with only two legs. And if you sit on a chair with two legs you're going to fall on your butt!

Just as a chair needs all four legs to support you, you need a complete and balanced approach to your health in order to sustain the results you are looking for.

The m.e.l.t approach to fitness is unique in that it is **balanced**. As is evident in our logo, there are four parts to m.e.l.t.; each of which is integrated with the others:

- The m.e.l.t. Mindset
- The m.e.l.t. Workout
- m.e.l.t. Meal Planning for Life
- The m.e.l.t. Lifestyle

The four parts of m.e.l.t. are here to help you achieve balanced health and fitness.

In this hectic world, it's too easy for certain aspects of our life, particularly work and family commitments, to spiral out of control. When that happens, your personal health and fitness is usually the first thing to get compromised. At m.e.l.t. we know that your health is the key to allowing you to successfully cope with the demands of work and home.

This book is about helping you achieve balance. If you're not a reader or are limited on time, just focus on reading a few sections every day. It's a quick read and you owe it to yourself to take the time to reflect and get inspired.

The biggest building in the world was built 1 brick at a time.

#justmelt

Joe Carabase
Creator of the m.e.l.t. Workout

M.E.L.T. PART 1: THE M.E.L.T. MINDSET

You are probably coming to m.e.l.t. with at least some prior experience in a big-box gym or with the latest-and-greatest exercise video sold from 3 a.m. infomercial. Maybe you tried P90X and it didn't work for you. Maybe you joined a $10/month facility filled with TVs, treadmills, and elliptical machines and it didn't work for you. **Just know that wasn't you who failed, it was the program that failed you.**

Those prior experiences brought you to m.e.l.t., and we're glad you're here! We want you to know that yes, you're going to see amazing results at m.e.l.t. You're going to get the body you want. But we also want to be clear that you've got to expect the unexpected along the way. And know that even after you hit your current goal, you will be reaching for others—goals you haven't even dreamed of yet. And each goal will be only part of the story that is going to be your fitness journey.

Every journey requires some preparation. At m.e.l.t., we think that the key to being successful starts with the following:

- Getting Your Mind Right
- Getting Your Goals Right

Getting Your Mind Right

All of our clients at m.e.l.t. — whether they're stay-at-home parents, business executives, normal nine-to-fivers, or students — have their own sets of challenges. Life is not easy, and at various points everyone faces challenging circumstances. We at m.e.l.t. know, and want you to know, that *challenges will happen.*

I think people go wrong when they expect fitness to be a straight line and they get started and, whether it's three months or 12 months, they're just going to do the program, get the result they want, and that will be the end of it. But that's not the way it works. **Fitness is not a destination, it's a lifelong journey**. And everything you do in your fitness life is only a chapter of your book of fitness. Every fitness journey has twists, turns, and unexpected roadblocks. If you're prepared for it to get a little crazy, you won't be thrown off when it happens.

Put On Your Own Oxygen Mask First

Do you have the tendency to put everyone else—kids, spouse, friends, job, family—ahead of yourself? On the surface, putting others first may sound like the right thing to do, but it's not.

The best example to illustrate this is the safety instructions found on every airline. In case of emergency, do airlines recommend you put the oxygen mask on your kid first or you?

You! Because taking care of your kid first would leave you gasping for air and create the need to help two people.

To be the person you want to be, to excel, and to help others around you, you need your health.

Putting on your own oxygen mask requires you to carve out time for yourself. Mark your calendars for when you m.e.l.t. and treat those times as if they're appointments you can't reschedule.

The Only Perfect Thing in Life is Taking Action

"Iteration is perfect."

I found this quote from entrepreneur Miki Agrawal interesting because it basically says the process is perfect. I'm a big believer that no one process is perfect, but I think the speaker is on to something here.

Your journey is perfect because it's imperfect— that makes sense right? I know this sounds silly, but hear me out.

There is no ONE perfect process. You can't do one program and expect everything to fall into place. Life is full of ups, downs, zig-zags, and pot holes you never see coming, all of which make sticking to a workout plan extremely difficult.

Realize that the true treasure is NOT 20 pounds lost or six-pack abs gained. The true treasure is *the journey you are on.*

Think about a day you don't feel like working out. If you are solely focused on the outcome you are seeking, you are of the mindset that anything less than 100 percent will be a failure. On the other hand, if you are focused on the process, all you need to do is put your shoes on and walk out the door and arrive at the gym.

You may not bring 100 percent, but if you bring 50 percent, that's 50 percent more than you would have brought otherwise. And over time, it adds up. *It's the workouts that you don't feel like doing that give you the greatest results.*

The only true perfect thing in life is taking action. Even a workout at 50 percent will make you feel better than you felt before. The better you feel after your workout, the more you will want to train. The more you train, the better you will look. The better you look and feel, the more you will want eat clean.

As Sir Isaac Newton stated:

An object in motion stays in motion … an object at rest stays at rest.

Remember that the journey won't always be pretty. There will be more days than not when you don't feel like training, so just put your shoes on and get yourself to your work out. There will be days where you have few options to eat right, so drink as much water as you can and make the best decisions with what you are given.

Just show up—you are always far more capable than you know.

How to Battle and Beat Your Inner Voice

Your inner voice can always justify doing something you know shouldn't.

- "Go ahead and have that last piece of pie—it's so small!"

- "You had such a hard day at work—give yourself a break and skip the workout!"

But just because your inner voice is giving you self-justifications, it doesn't mean you have to listen! You can fight back—and here's how:

1. **All change starts with awareness.** Start noticing when you make self- justifications. I recommend writing these reasons down or putting them in your phone's note pad.
2. **Go 30 miles per hour.** If 0 mph is eating and drinking whatever you want on the weekend and 60 mph is

drinking water and eating plain chicken/eggs/broccoli all weekend, 30 mph would be having a cheat meal and not drinking OR having a drink with a salad.

3. **Forgive yourself.** You can't be "on" all the time—no one is. Chalk up going off plan as fuel instead of as a loss. For instance, yesterday I had an extra serving of dessert for my little nephew Jesse's birthday. So now I will just prolong my fast tomorrow and I'll work even harder in my workout.

4. **F.O.C.U.S.** *"Follow One Path Until Success."* In a complex world**, simplicity** wins every time. I can tell you that looking at every situation with F.O.C.U.S. and simplicity has made me less stressed and more productive. This is still something I am working on, but the more I practice it, the better everything becomes. Self-justification LOVES when you have a million things going on because it's just more excuses you have available. Remove clutter to think clearly.

5. **Talk back.** When the voice says you're too tired to m.e.l.t. and you'll start tomorrow, *talk back*! Tell the voice it's only 30 minutes and that you will feel awesome and proud for going.

6. **Remember, you're not alone.** Everyone in the #meltfamily goes through this sort of thing, and we've got your back.

Self-Doubt is Self-Made

At certain points in your fitness journey, you may start to question why you ever got started in the beginning--and if it's worth all the work to continue. Look, if you don't ever question yourself than you are not human. Self-doubt and negative talk are part of our genetic makeup. It's not the end of the world to feel self-doubt – what's more important is how you respond. Do you let the negativity overpower you? Or do you hold your ground, stay positive and keep moving forward?

You've heard the quote and it's true: "If you say you can, you are right. If you say you cannot, you are also right."

So STOP with the negatives —"I can't ... I won't ... I'll try ..."—there is NO try.

You either do or don't. When you start our m.e.l.t. program, you are not trying, you are doing! This mind shift is huge because you are acknowledging progress. And progress breeds more progress.

Get Your Win In

You can immediately improve how your day is going by chalking up a win. What constitutes a win? Anything positive that brings you closer to your goal, or things that make you feel good after the fact. Eating a chocolate might make you feel good initially, but not so much an hour later.

The other day a group of our #meltfamily was m.e.l.t.ing it forward at the St. Jude's Walk and I saw one of our Rock Stars, Michelle, who lost more than 100 pounds since joining in April, take down a small yet extremely effective win. There was a "VIP tent" where we could get free food and snacks for helping. They had these cookies that the old Michelle used to LOVE.

What did she do?

She chose an apple instead – a win! And then she came over

to talk to me about it –another win! The latter is not a win because she told me—it has nothing to do with me. The win is that she shared a story about how she was emotionally tied to those cookies, how hard it was for her not to grab one, but yet she still made the right decision in grabbing the apple.

These small wins are simple things yet reveal a lot of baggage; for example, Michelle's personal attachment to the cookies. Another example of baggage we see all the time is when people had a bad experience with another boot camp, gym, trainer, or DVD and are now afraid to even step foot into m.e.l.t. OR pop in our DVD. The win in this case would be just showing up: we will take it from there. But the previous experience can be heavy baggage.

Personally I know if I don't work out that I don't feel as good about myself either, but I know if I can score a few wins, I'll feel much better. Here are my top three go-tos:

1. MOVE! Whether I am sick, too tired, too sore, or too busy, I know that it will help to just do a few movements, no matter how basic.

2. Talk to someone in the #meltfamily in person or on the phone (one of my team members or m.e.l.t.ers).

3. Make someone smile.

Our most successful m.e.l.t.ers implement our "progress NOT perfection" motto by working in the following quick self-improvement wins that take only minutes:

1. Just show up at m.e.l.t.

2. Read even just a couple of pages of any self-development book (personal, business, or health)

3. Drink water throughout the day, aiming for .55 times your bodyweight in ounces of water per day

4. Bring your lunch to work

5. Park further away

6. Introduce yourself to someone new who might be timid or nervous

7. Get outside your comfort zone—even doing just one more rep than you think you can do

8. Put down the fork when you're satisfied

9. Walk past the candy jar or tray of cookies at work

10. Choose the healthier menu option

11. Take 60 seconds and doing one stretch that makes you feel good

12. Roll the bottom of your foot (or any other part of your body) as you are talking with your co-worker, significant other, and/or kids

13. After you brush your teeth immediately upon waking, crush a 30-second plank. Just make sure to brush first so you don't knock yourself out with stank breath. (I'm

not saying you in particular have bad breath but you know the whole morning breath thing and in a plank position you are face to face with the floor!)

14. Put your m.e.l.t. meal plan on your refrigerator

15. Randomly drop and do as many push-ups as you can (Google "Joe Carabase Batmanning" for a fun video) OR if you don't feel like pushing it, drop and do five push-ups—I KNOW you have five push-ups inside you!

16. Put your m.e.l.t. books, deck of cards, or any other workout-related books around the house where you'll see them. Seeing is motivating!

    Side note: Seeing can be demotivating as well. One of the worst things you can have in the bedroom is that darn treadmill which is now an expensive clothes hanger. Each day you're reminded of not using it, for which I don't blame you because it's boring and not as effective.

17. Go for a five-minute walk before you eat your lunch.

18. Put your goal statement on your bathroom mirror where you can see it first thing. Tape a note, your m.e.l.t. workout calendar to it or write on it with a dry erase marker—it doesn't matter how, just get that goal in your face

19. Watch TV as you roll your left glute (a.k.a. "butt cheek") for 30 seconds before switching to the other.

20. Fill in the blank—can be anything that will help support your goal

As motivational speaker Les Brown says, *you can't stroll your goal!* You can't just expect to see what you want to see by doing little or nothing at all. Find ways to fit in those workout chunks to make your fitness a lifestyle. I guarantee you'll start amazing yourself!

How to Get on SportsCenter Top 10 Plays

Don't try to get on ESPN's SportsCenter Top 10 Plays!

While it might be glamorous to focus on dazzling changes like the five-pound drop on the scale in one week, remember that these are just small parts of the entire game. The SportsCenter highlight of the awesome play that took only 10 seconds is only possible because of the other 59 minutes and 50 seconds, on top of the entire off-season of work.

Personally, I made this mistake early on in my career as a fitness entrepreneur. Out of college, I had this vision of what my gym would look like, being on TV and getting national recognition for helping people. But the problem was I didn't deserve to achieve any of those things. I use to get frustrated wondering why those things weren't happening, and I spent a lot of energy on this frustration until one day my mentor Paul Reddick set me straight. He opened my eyes to how selfish I was being. I was focusing on the wrong things and taking away from the energy I could be giving to help more people.

While I still set breakthrough goals, I shifted my energy towards what I can do for others day to day. Since doing this, so many of the things I've dreamed about have come true—becoming a regular on NBC Connecticut and Better Connecticut, becoming a top-three finalist for *Men's Health* Next Top Trainer and getting sought out for advice and speaking from peers across the country. But most important, I've been able to make a greater impact on more people.

If you want to make a greater impact on your body, job, or life, focus your energy on the day-to-day grind.

And acknowledge every small bit of progress. Otherwise, it will be forgotten and you will wrongly think you're stuck. But sometimes you can't see progress. Believe that the small progress you're making every day will get you to where you want to be.

The m.e.l.t. Motto: Progress, Not Perfection

We have a saying here at m.e.l.t.: Progress, not perfection. We don't believe in perfect. We believe in perfect effort. Because we know that if you are putting in the right amount of effort, in our program, we will always see results. The reality is that if your goal is weight loss and you're just looking at the scale, then what you think is going to be progress is when that scale goes down. However, that doesn't show you how strong you got, how much better you can move. It doesn't show how you feel. It doesn't show the inches off your waist. In that setting, that might be a plateau for you if you're just looking at the scale. However, when you're measuring the things that matter, things that you can measure accurately—which is not the scale but things such as inches off your waist or performance of a movement—then in a program like m.e.l.t., you literally will never plateau.

Our workouts will always challenge you in different ways so that your body is forced to adapt or is forced to get stronger because it can never adapt. We have a three-week phase—throughout those three weeks, Monday through Saturday changes every week. Every week builds off the previous week. Every phase builds off the previous phase. So, your body is going to be presented with new challenges and it takes time to change, but over time, you will progress and get better.

Would You Compare Yourself to a Tree?

I highly doubt it. Why? Because a tree is not a human and comparing yourself to a tree seems silly and useless. But honestly it's not much different than you comparing yourself to another human.

You literally create impossible standards for yourself when you compare yourself to others because you're not making an even comparison. Comparing yourself to anyone else is truly an apples-to-oranges comparison. Yes, both apples and oranges are food. Yes, you and that woman in the yoga pants at Starbucks are both human. Cool! But that is where the fair comparisons end.

At our First Annual m.e.l.t.ys (which was an amazing night, by the way), I had the opportunity to speak to many m.e.l.t.ers and hear about their incredible stories.

One of our Simsbury Rock Stars, Rosie, said something that I found extremely inspirational. Rosie has lost over 80 pounds and if you looked at her "before" picture, you would not believe it was her. She's now confident, lean, and firm from head to toe.

Rosie said she was hesitant to post her "before" pictures but did so because she wanted people to see her both then and now, and to know that transformation is possible.

How often do you look at someone and just assume that person has it good? That he or she has been fit all their life and that it just comes easy to them? I'll admit I've been guilty of that myself.

But the fact is we have no idea what the story is with that person. Maybe, like Rosie, they were once 80 pounds overweight. Maybe they dedicate themselves to m.e.l.t.ing six times per week and eating clean 80 percent of the time, year-round. Maybe they've had surgery done or have taken performance enhancers.

The bottom line is, YOU NEVER KNOW SOMEONE'S BACK STORY—AND WE ALL HAVE ONE.

And you know that cover model? Let me tell you from experience, she does not look like that from day to day. In most cases, looking like a cover model requires extreme dieting, a lot of makeup, and plenty of Photoshop retouching.

So the best and only comparison to make is YOU vs. YOU. And the best way to measure your progress is to take a picture of yourself in a bathing suit and compare the image every 49 days. Why 49 days? We've found it's the shortest amount of time to make the biggest type of transformation.

To accurately judge your progress, you have to measure things like:

- **Body composition** – using "before" and "after" pictures
- **Circumference measurements** – waist, hips, thighs, and upper arms
- **Performance** – stability, strength, and endurance

When you compare your current self to your former self, you start to unleash your 20X factor—the realization that you can do 20 times more than you currently think you are capable of.

And you know what we say about progress—Progress Breeds Progress!

No one else in the world is as amazing and as awesome as you are; you can't argue this point—it's time for YOU to start to own it. Trust me, when you do BIG transformations, it will start happening physically, emotionally, and spiritually.

20X More Capability Than You Think

Through studying human performance and what humans are actually capable of, the Navy SEALs have discovered that each of us, including you, has 20 times (20X) the capability inside us than we currently think. This means that regardless of whatever you think you can do right now, you can do 20X more.

After the m.e.l.t. MS charity workout in Glastonbury last fall, it was time for burpee pledges - $5 for 5 burpees. I was pledging my team and myself, and members were pledging each other as well as coaches for reasonable amounts of burpees.

And just when we thought it was over, m.e.l.t Rock Star Heather Mitchell pledged me $100 for 100 burpees! What a doll, eh?

What's important for you to understand here is that I have never done 100 consecutive burpees, nor had I been training to do 100 consecutive burpees. If someone had asked how many burpees I could do in a row, I have no idea what I would have said, but it wouldn't have been close to 100.

We ALL underestimate our abilities and put limitations on ourselves.

The reality is that you can do 99 percent of most things: dropping 20 pounds, performing push-ups or pull-ups for reps, running a Spartan race, or crushing our m.e.l.t. boot camp workout six days a week. Yet often just because you haven't done something before, you think or say you *can't*.

If you haven't done something before, how do know you can't do it? Don't get stuck in the trap of confusing self-imposed limitations with factual evidence.

If Heather had pledged 100 burpees a week before the charity workout, I would have thought about it for a week. The more you think about something, the more overwhelming that something becomes. In this case, I had no choice but to just get it done. Remember, there is no try. If you want something, go for it now because the longer you wait the harder it will be.

Once you become a m.e.l.t.er, we hook you up with a "team m.e.l.t. and 20x" bracelet to remind you, during those moments of weakness, that you have more in the tank.

Every Step Forward is Progress

Whatever your goal is that you are seeking, just go for it. Realize that things might not go exactly to plan but that it *will* work out in the end if you keep pressing forward. Every step forward is progress, even if it doesn't look like it.

Don't get paralyzed by the "what if's" and the previous workout programs/diets that have failed you. To find your way, all you have to do is "do"—just m.e.l.t. You can't reach the summit without first climbing the mountain.

When it comes to your workouts, just show up and we'll coach you from there. Just buy healthier foods. Just eat fewer processed foods and drink more water. As you'll see with the m.e.l.t. meal plan, eating clean is actually just as simple as eating poorly—you just have to decide which you want.

Throughout this process remember you are above average. Napoleon Hill (considered one of the great writers on personal success) found that less than four percent of people do extraordinary things, that most people live just average lives. The expectation is average or even worse. But here's the thing—YOU are ABOVE average. How do I know? Because you (we) were designed with more ability than we could ever realize in one lifetime. And the fact that you're reading this means you are looking to unleash more of that ability.

It's Literally This Simple

There is no pill or magic wand that will make you lose fat. But losing fat fast is not rocket science, either. You already have everything you need to make it happen, despite what others have told you and what you've told yourself about past experiences. m.e.l.t. is the one program that is designed to work for you no matter your fitness level or how busy your life is.

Let's get you in the best possible shape—FAST. Here are 9 things you can do to help:

1. **Just show up** – The hardest part is either showing up at m.e.l.t. or popping the m.e.l.t. At Home DVD in. Once you're there or it's in, we got you.

2. **Get comfortable getting uncomfortable** – It's not supposed to be easy!

3. **Affirm yourself daily** – "*Every Day in Every Way I Am Getting Better and Better*"

4. **Drink more water** – .55 times your weight in ounces of water per day

5. **Schedule your workouts** – Carve out at least three m.e.l.t. workouts each week. Write them down and treat your m.e.l.t. workout like any other important appointment.

6. **Get ready to get back up quickly** – You will be misdirected, things will not always go to plan, and you will stumble. Get back up, keep moving forward.

7. **Roll your body tissues daily** – Using a foam roller or a tennis ball, lacrosse ball, or softball

8. **Eat fewer processed foods** – Start kicking the crap out of your diet and keep eliminating those additive-laden foods. Eat lean, eat clean!

9. **Empower others** – Someone close to you is watching. Lead by example.

Getting Your Goals Right

We talked earlier about one of our Rock Stars, Michelle. She was overweight, and literally in seven months, she has lost more than 120 pounds, just by doing the workouts and following her diet. There's no starvation, no pills, no surgery. She did that just through hard work in our program. Now, even with Michelle, she's at a point where she's not seeing much of a change on the scale. And that happens in every weight loss journey. She's lost so much excess body fat and weight, but now she's increasing her lean muscle. There's a point where your scale is not going to move because you've lost most of your extra weight. While you can still maybe lose a few pounds, the fitter you get, the harder it will be for you to see a change on the scale. The lean muscle percent is going to increase, and muscle weighs more than fat. So it's not going to show up on a scale.

So yes, it's good to have weight loss goals if they're realistic, but just understand that at a certain point, those goals will become obsolete. So we always like to have an additional goal besides weight loss—tangible goals you can measure—something like fitting into those jeans that maybe you haven't fit into since before your kid was born or running a 5K or doing a push-up. Anything performance-wise, and it really can be anything, or any clothes to fit into, but it's important to have an exact thing you can measure. Because the difference between fitting into those jeans and losing 20 pounds is that you can actively measure the distance, the difference on your waist. You can literally take a circumference measurement and you can see.

You can't see the change necessarily in weight loss, because at all times during the m.e.l.t. workout, you're going to be building lean muscle. Don't let that scare you, because lean muscle is going to help you get toned up and help you burn body fat.

You can see it, but you can't measure it when you're stepping on a scale—how much is lean muscle, how much is body fat? So you have no way of knowing. If the scale doesn't change, it might tell you that, and it's easy for you to think that you're not getting anywhere. However, that doesn't mean that you're not building muscle and it doesn't mean that you're not getting fitter. So it's just not a good goal to look at.

What is Your "Why?"

When you find a meaningful "why" for a particular goal, you create a powerful tool that will help propel you forward and keep you going when it gets tough.

The most important thing for all of us to understand is that it's not just about losing weight or fitting into those jeans. There are deep psychological reasons as to why.

It's important to figure out the "why" because when you can link goals to your deep personal desires, you'll do whatever you can to make sure those things are met. They always say that you'll work harder for someone else than you will for yourself. And oftentimes, that somebody else is either physically somebody else—like your kids or your parents or your significant other—or sometimes it's that person inside of you that you haven't met yet because she/he has been buried with self-doubt and bad experiences and being overweight.

So you say, "Okay, I want to lose weight." To get to the real reason for wanting it, you need to keep digging. Set an alarm for 10 minutes and just keep writing the reasons that come to mind as you think about why you want to lose weight. After you write down each reason, ask yourself "*What's so important about that?"* and write down your answer. This process will help you dig deep.

The first reasons you write will be more superficial—like they could apply to anyone. But the more you continue to "peel back the onion" the deeper, more emotional reasons you will uncover. There are no right or wrong answers because it's your personal experience. The goal is to find the deepest emotional reasoning. How will you know once you found it? **You will feel the emotion associated with it.**

Here's an example of "peeling back the onion":

- **I want to lose weight.**

  What's so important about that?

- **I want to fit into my skinny jeans again.**

  What's so important about that?

- **I want to wear fashionable clothes.**

  What's so important about that?

- **I will feel better about myself.**

  What's so important about that?

- **My confidence will increase.**

  What's so important about that?

- **I can be the positive example my kids need.**

  What's so important about that?

- **I will set the right foundation for them so they can grow up with self-confidence and not have to deal**

with what I went through as kid.

So which goal do you think is more powerful?

A. Lose weight.

B. Set the right foundation for my kids so they can grow up with self-confidence and not deal with what I went through as kid.

The idea is that you're continually taking what you have as a goal, whatever comes to mind, and you're peeling it back like an onion where your end goal is nothing like the first goal you gave.

So remember, you need to dig deep to find your "why." Getting to the core of your "why" will give you an important tool you need to reach your goals. To uncover your deepest emotional wants and needs, you have to keep answering the question, "Why?" The more you ask yourself why, the more you will write, and the deeper you will get.

It's Time for You to Get Real

One of the benefits of setting and writing down goals is that when you do so, you program your subconscious mind, which is more powerful than our conscious mind, to will automatically act in your favor. Regardless of whether or not you know your subconscious mind exists and you actually use it in your favor, it will work for or against you, based on the things you're writing down, based on the things you're saying. So when it comes to goal setting, you can actively take charge of your subconscious mind by writing down specifically what you want to happen, and talking in terms of it happening—things like "I will," or, "I cannot wait until …"

Talk about the feelings you will have once you reach those goals. When you do that, you start to create awareness in your subconscious mind of whatever your goals are. And this is important because now you have something working for you, an amazing power that's working for you when you're not thinking about it.

Just Do What Bruce Lee and Jim Carrey Did!

There's a lot for us to learn from top performers and actors. I think we all have the tendency to look at celebrities and believe that success came easily to them. We assume they had the right connections, got really lucky, or they were just born naturally talented. But Jim Carrey and Bruce Lee wouldn't be where they are today if they didn't set challenging goals and then use their goals as inspiration to work their butts off.

As a struggling comedian in 1990, Jim Carrey wrote a blank check for $10 million to himself for acting services. While that check wasn't real, it was something visual he used to program his mind for the success he wanted to achieve.

Before Bruce Lee ever got into a movie, he wrote, "By 1980, I will be the best-known Oriental movie star in the United States and will have secured $10 million." At that time, he had very little acting experience, but he had the body, he had the capability, and he had the desire. He wrote his goal down and then he worked to get it.

How can you keep your own goals in the forefront of your mind? If your goal is to fit back into a favorite pair of jeans, you could hang them in your bathroom or somewhere you're going to see them every single day. Those jeans will remind you of your goal, and inspire you to work to achieve it.

You Are a Work of Art in Progress

Let's imagine we had a time machine. Would you have the nerve to go back in time to 1508 when Michelangelo started painting the ceiling of the Sistine Chapel, look over his back, and critique his effort?

No way. At least not knowing what a masterpiece the ceiling evolved into.

How is this any different from you getting down on yourself because you don't lose three pounds a week every week? Or because you've been working out for two months and haven't lost 20 pounds?

You are a masterpiece in progress. No body transformation is too large or small—you can get the body you want.

The problem with solely focusing on an outcome is that it's extremely hard to measure along the way, especially when it comes to weight loss. If you're weighing yourself weekly, you are setting yourself up for failure, as the scale simply is not the best measure of real progress. Real progress is not only pounds lost.

Another problem with outcome-based goals is that they're not actionable—how do you know where to start? I could have the goal of climbing a mountain, but if I don't know the path, I'm screwed!

Now is the perfect time to sit down and write what you will look like one year from today. Notice I wrote "will," not "want to." Wanting and wishing are for fairy tales. When you declare "you will" do something, it becomes real.

Being as specific as possible, write down what your waist measurement will be, how your arms will look, how your legs will look, the types of clothes you will wear, what your weight will be, how your significant other will look at you, and so on. Don't hold back—get it ALL down!

Then write down how you will measure your success. The best ways to do this are:

- The number of workouts—both boot camp and at-home—you will crush each week
- How many clean meals/snacks you will eat per week
- How many cheat meals you will allow per month
- How many push-ups you will do in a row—and other similar performance-based goals, such as lunges, squats, and burpees

While none of these goals directly correlates to weight loss or inches off, they are the benchmarks you need to focus on to see the weight and inches literally m.e.l.t. off.

The funny thing about goals is when you write them down, they actually happen—which is another important reason to focus on the process. If you spend all of your energy on losing the 20 pounds (the outcome), what happens when you lose the 20 pounds? Too often, people suffer from fear of success, and one of the reasons is because they don't know what to do when they get there. When you focus on the process, the goal doesn't matter. You can use the same process over and over again.

We are so lucky to wake up every day and step out of bed—

there are people out there who would give their left arm to do that.

This next year will not be easy. But you have more than everything you need to battle whatever obstacles get thrown in your way.

Remember, you are a work of art in progress. And YOU hold the paint brush.

Got TOMA?

TOMA, or Top-Of-Mind Awareness, is an ally in your journey towards getting the body you want. When you take your goals out of your head and write them down, they become real. And when you keep those written goal near you—in your wallet, on your bathroom mirror, in your car, in your office, or anywhere else—and reread them frequently during the day, the more you are reminded of and inspired to achieve them. **That's top-of-mind awareness. What we think about is what we become.**

One of the things you've got to understand is that the journey to your goal is not linear. It's not straight. It's messy. It's curvy. It's winding. Things rarely go according to your plan. So, your goals might change. Maybe you set lofty goals and it turns out you don't quite reach them but you come close—that's fine. You probably came closer than you would have otherwise. Or maybe you set goals that were too small and you blew them out of the water. So you've got to actively set your goals, actively reflect upon them, and know that the path to achieving them is not going to be a perfectly straight line. Things will get a little messy at times, but if you follow this process, you have no worries.

Progress is Not Linear

Your fitness journey can be messy. There are obstacles. There are distractions. There are detours. There will be rainy days. You know this. Don't let it bring you down, but don't be surprised when it shows up. And when it shows up, you've got to focus on persisting and moving forward.

If you miss your workout, the best way to keep moving forward is to schedule your next workout. When you eat outside of your meal plan—and sometimes you don't expect it and it just happens, for whatever reason—focus on planning your very next meal or snack. When you can do this, you lift yourself up and you continue moving forward. When you hiccup by missing a workout, it's only bad if you don't make the next step forward in the right direction. Because you're either going forward or backward, right? So if you don't step forward after that, then that means you're retracting. And this is where most people fall, because there's a chain reaction. Momentum builds momentum, and progress breeds progress. If you can continue on your path toward your goals, then even if you get sidetracked, you can get right back onto that path and you'll get to where you want to go. But if you let one thing happen and then the next thing happen, before you know it two weeks have passed. Then it's three months and all of your hard work has gone away just because of that one first mistake. So persist when things go wrong--because something always will--and just get back on track and you'll get exactly where you want to go.

We run two seven-week challenges every year. One seven-week challenge is during a very hectic time of year—the transition from back-to-school to the holidays. That's a time when many people give up their fitness goals and say, "You know what, too much going on. I'm going to get started in January." And then when January rolls around, they're 10 pounds heavier than where they were before.

One of our m.e.l.t. clients, who knew she was going to be travelling frequently during the challenge, decided to sign up anyway. She said, "You know what? I'm still going to do it, I'm going to stay the course and follow the program." Well, not only did she travel, she got sick. And then her kids got sick. But she never quit. She kept moving forward. At the end of the seven weeks, she lost 14 pounds and many inches off her stomach. To me, that was the biggest transformation of the challenge, because her journey was not straight at all; she had a lot of roadblocks put in her way. Many people quit under the least duress and say, "You know what? I tried. Whatever." But she didn't. She kept going forward. She persisted. She leveraged the workout plan and she had results to show for it.

M.E.L.T. PART 2: THE M.E.L.T. WORKOUT

More than Just a Gym

Most people think of working out as a chore, but when you come to m.e.l.t., you get to escape from the outside world with its negativity or stress and focus on the most important thing—you. No drama, no getting yelled at, no boring cardio, no standing around waiting for an exercise machine or feeling pressured to look good or get dressed up for the workouts—NO expectations you have to meet except for just showing up.

Why You'll Feel Good When You Come to M.E.L.T.

Our members have told us countless times that the way the m.e.l.t. experience makes them feel is what motivates them make time in their schedule and push themselves to the limit. When you come to m.e.l.t. you will feel comfortable because:

- You will be warmly welcomed by the #meltfamily (m.e.l.t. team and members) the second you walk in. The comfort you feel allows you to settle your nerves and anxiety. In a normal gym setting, these two things can drain you more than your actual workout.

- Everyone works within his or her own level, which removes the pressure for you to compete but makes you want to work harder because each person is working hard within his or her fitness level.

- You belong to something bigger then yourself. People count on you showing up and actually care if you do or don't.

- There are only good and great workouts at m.e.l.t.—NEVER bad workouts. You will always feel better leaving than you did coming in and because of this you will not want to miss your workouts.

When you feel comfortable and when you feel good, you'll find a way to be here. As you know, this is the most difficult challenge when it comes to fitness. And once you're here, we'll coach you to where you want to be.

The M.E.L.T. Minimum

Nowadays people are training too hard for too long. They force themselves to endure 45+ minute workouts that cause their body to break down and that lead to injury or inability to sleep (another sign of overtraining).

m.e.l.t. workouts are designed for the minimum dosage of exercise you need to maximize results, to never plateau, and to avoid the risk of over-training.

It's not about how long you work out or how many workouts you do in a day, it's about the intensity you bring and the effectiveness of the program you train within. **Research proves that the number-one indicator of getting the results you want is intensity, not duration.** By working out at a high intensity with short rest periods, your body post-exercise continues to need oxygen at a higher rate, raising your metabolic rate for up to 48 hours.

What You Can Expect at M.E.L.T.

- **Fun-Friendly Atmosphere:** There's ZERO judging and TONS of support from both fellow m.e.l.t.ers and your coaches. **You'll walk out happier and more energized every time!**

- **High Tempo for <u>ALL FITNESS LEVELS</u>:** The m.e.l.t. Workout is unlike anything you've experienced. While it is fast paced, it's NOT all high impact, and we accommodate all fitness levels at once. For your first few weeks, focus on mastering the level-one exercises.

- **Self-Massage**: We highly encourage you to come five to 10 minutes early to foam roll to relieve muscular tension and increase mobility. A coach or fellow m.e.l.t.er will take you through how to foam roll when you get here, but basically you just want to put the implement (foam roller, lacrosse ball, or softball) above or below major joints (ankle, knee, hip, shoulder) and apply your body pressure to roll in tense areas. We recommend you do also do this at home.

- **Progress Every Week:** The m.e.l.t. Workout is on a three-week phase where the six workouts (Monday through Saturday) progress from the previous week.

- **Predictable Results**: *No more guessing how hard to train!* m.e.l.t. has a state-of-the-art heart rate monitoring system that allows you to see the percentage of your max heart rate and calories burned at all times. When you get a heart rate monitor, the coach can advise you what heart rate percent you should be training at, based on your goals.

Let m.e.l.t. Work for You Rather than You for It

m.e.l.t.30 is about leveraging time to get you the best possible result.

A flaw of most other workout programs is that they are too long. This leads to overtraining, potential injury, and diminishing results. In long workouts, you are unable to efficiently reach the "edge" or the point where you are working as hard as you can outside your comfort zone. The shorter period of time until you reach this edge, the harder your body has to work to recover, thus increasing your post-metabolic rate. In traditional long workouts, the edge is not reached until 45 to 60 minutes later, which has a small impact on your resting metabolic rate. In these m.e.l.t. workouts, you'll achieve the "edge" in half the time of traditional workouts, allowing you to get more done in less time.

The hardest part in the m.e.l.t. program is just showing up. It's walking through those doors. It's just finding a way to get there, because you've got so much going on in your life. Just getting to m.e.l.t. or popping in the m.e.l.t. DVD—that is the hardest part. Because once you're there, we'll take care of the rest. Our program is designed to give you the biggest result in the shortest amount of time. Everything you do, every second of the 30-minute workout, is programmed to maximize your time spent and to make sure that you never plateau. Simply show up and you are already leveraging everything you can.

We live in a society that teaches us that *more is better* but this is not the case when it comes to m.e.l.t. Workouts. Sure, coming in 6 days per week would be more beneficial than 3 days per week. However, for these workouts to be as effective as they're designed, you need to *give everything you have* in each workout. That's why we don't allow you to take multiple classes per day –

it would be a waste of time. If you could do two m.e.l.t. classes in a day, then you're not putting in enough effort into each class. How do we know? Because there is endless progressions to each movement inside every m.e.l.t. workout and if you're going 100%, you should be completely fatigued. While you might be able to get away with this for a short period of time, you eventually will over train and the results you seek will start to diminish.

Two-a-day training is popular in the bodybuilding world so that you can focus on multiple parts of the body with ample energy supply. But body building is not m.e.l.t.ing. While there are several components of bodybuilding (muscle definition, toning) inside of our workouts, bodybuilding workouts are longer & lower intensity by nature so more time can be spent on developing muscle size & distinction to develop overall symmetry. If your goal is not to get on a stage, bodybuilding type workouts will not be beneficial to you.

How much should you do in addition to m.e.l.t.ing?

One side effect of these workouts is that you're going to be feeling really good about yourself and will want to do more. That's great but again you want to make sure you are putting all your energy in the 30-minute workout. Outside of that you shouldn't have much extra to spare. The most resistance-based type workout you could add to your day would be a 5-minute density set (yes, five minutes only) but it should be the opposite of your m.e.l.t. Workout. For example, if you train in the am, the 5-min density set should be in the pm.

During our challenges and transformation contests, we provide a 30-30-30 and various other quick sets that are good to add to your routine. The 30-30-30 is 30 push-ups, 30 burpees, and 30 squats performed as fast as you can with good form.

Remember that these sets are most effective when you can do them opposite or away from your m.e.l.t. Workouts so you can bring more intensity to them, which translates into greater results. If you put in 100% during your m.e.l.t. workout, after the finisher you should be toast!

How Much Weight Should You Use?

Think of "light" as something you can use to perform most movements 12 or more reps. Think of "heavy" as something you can only perform most movements for six to 12 reps.

Maximum Muscle Growth – 6-12 reps: For people whose goals are to get stronger and build as much lean muscle as possible. Note that you will still be burning body fat.

Muscular Endurance – 12 plus reps: For people who primarily want to build lean muscle and lose weight. Note that you shouldn't be doing more than 30 reps, so if you can easily do 15 reps of something, the weight is too light.

What is The M.E.L.T. Routine?

The m.e.l.t. philosophy was created to deliver an all-encompassing routine that fuses together the best of each of discipline; the definition and toning of bodybuilding, the afterburn fat loss from your metabolism, the respiratory endurance from cardio, strength training, stability and function from core training, mobility and flexibility from power yoga, and non-traditional—fun effective movements from underground training.

Each workout within each phase progresses in difficulty each week, and is designed to accelerate your results. For best results, we recommend you pick the specific days you want to attend and attend those throughout our three-week phase. You will build mastery of movement through the three-week phase, which will allow you to achieve a greater result.

Monday: Lower Body Cardio Strengthening

This workout is a strength-based workout. For best results and ONLY after you feel comfortable with your form, we recommend you choose a higher weight for lower reps. This means you will have to pause in between reps or even drop the weight for a few seconds within the set. This is okay as long as you keep going forward.

A good indication of poor form with lower body movements is feeling low back pain. This results in either rounded shoulders, not firing the right muscles and/or tight hamstrings and glutes. If you feel any low back pain, let a coach know immediately!

ALWAYS start with light weight and progress to heavier once your form is locked in.

Tuesday & Thursday: m.e.l.t.ABOLIC

This workout is geared towards fat loss and afterburn training. Basically, how hard you go during the work sets will dictate how many calories you burn at rest. Once you lock in your form, go as hard as you can during the given work set for best results.

We recommend you start moving slower and only progress to faster once your form is locked in.

Wednesday: Upper Body Cardio Strengthening

Just like the lower body workout, this is a strength-based workout, so choose a heavier weight—again only after you lock in your form.

ALWAYS start with light weight and progress to heavier once

your form is locked in.

Friday: Abs Sculpting

This total core workout is designed to give you stability, improve posture, remove low back pain, and help you get a tighter tummy. During this workout, focus on squeezing both your glutes and your stomach. Imagine that you were holding a $100 bill between your butt cheeks—you want to lock it in! With your stomach, imagine someone was punching you and you were bracing by sucking your stomach in towards your spinal cord.

Saturday: m.e.l.t.ed Cardio

Also known as "adult recess," this workout will get you moving in all different directions, and increase your aerobic capacity. It's very important here that you start moving slow and only progress to faster movement once you feel comfortable with the movement.

What Workouts Should You Do?

Another unique feature of the m.e.l.t. Workout is that you can train six days a week without over-training because each day has a specific focus, which allows other parts of your body to rest.

We don't recommend the number of days based on your fitness level, but rather on how many days you can commit to. We want to set you up for success, and we know that if you come here you will see amazing results, but getting here is the hardest part.

With that said, based on your goals, here are some baseline recommendations. There is no wrong choice because **ALL** m.e.l.t. workouts will give you great benefits!

Beginner

People who are currently working out fewer than three times

per week on a consistent basis. We define a consistent basis as something you have done for three or more consecutive months. This is the perfect starting point for people who have been too busy to work out and stick to the traditional workout routine.

- If you are concerned about losing weight, focus on coming Tuesday, Thursday, and Friday. Focus on keeping your heart rate at 70 to 80 percent of your max heart rate for most of the workout. If you see it slowing down and you're comfortable with your form, aim for higher reps. When you find yourself more comfortable, focus on keeping your heart rate at 83 to 88 percent of your max heart rate most the workout. Let it go during the finisher—aim to be in the red (over 88 percent).

- If you are concerned with toning up and building strength, focus on Monday, Wednesday, and Friday. Focus on keeping your heart rate at 65 to 78% of your max heart rate for most of the workout. If you see it jumping up, slow down and use heavier weight. Focus on keeping your heart rate at 78 to 83% of your max heart rate for most of the workout. Let it go during the finisher—aim to be in the red (over 88 percent).

*If you can commit to coming more days per week, you will see greater results. Again, it's not a matter of if you can come more often from a physical ability perspective as much as it's if you can make it work in your schedule.

Intermediate

People who are currently working out three or more times per week on a consistent basis.

- If you are concerned about losing weight, focus on

coming Tuesday, Thursday, Friday, Saturday, and Monday OR Wednesday, based on whichever you would consider your weak point, lower body or upper body. Focus on keeping your heart rate at 83 to 88 percent of your max heart rate for most of the workout. If you see it slowing down and you're comfortable with your form, aim for higher reps. Give it your all during the finisher—aim to be in the red (over 90 percent).

- If you are concerned with toning up and building strength, focus on Monday, Tuesday, or Thursday (doesn't matter which day), Wednesday, Friday, and Saturday. Focus on keeping your heart rate at 78 to 83 percent of your max heart rate for most of the workout. If you see it jumping up, slow down and use heavier weight. However, let it go during the finisher—aim to be in the red (over 90 percent).

Advanced

People who are currently working out five or more times per week on a consistent basis. We recommend that you m.e.l.t. six days per week to achieve your ultimate potential. During each workout, continually focus on keeping your heart rate within the appropriate ranges based on your goals:

- If you are concerned about losing weight, focus on coming Tuesday, Thursday, Friday, Saturday, and Monday OR Wednesday, based on whichever you would consider your weak point, lower body or upper body. Focus on keeping your heart rate at 83 to 88 percent of your max heart rate for most of the workout. If you see it slowing down and you're comfortable with your form, aim for higher reps. Let it go during the finisher—aim to be in the red (over 90 percent).

- If you are concerned with toning up and building strength, focus on Monday, Tuesday, or Thursday (doesn't matter which day), Wednesday, Friday, and Saturday. Focus on keeping your heart rate at 78 to 83 percent of your max heart rate for most of the workout. If you see it jumping up, slow down and use heavier weight. However, let it go during the finisher—aim to be in the red (over 90 percent).

What You Should Feel When M.E.L.T.ing

You should aim to train at a level that challenges you within the heart rate zones that fit within your goals. For example, you should not be able to hold a conversation with someone. Do not train to failure or past exhaustion. Remember, you can always take a few seconds off during the workout, just stay with your group and rotate as they rotate.

Stop training and let a coach know immediately if you:

- Feel nauseous
- Light-headed
- Dizzy
- Are sweating excessively
- Feel extreme skin temperature change
- Experience anything else that does not feel right

Listen to YOUR body.

If something feels wrong, stop immediately and wave over a coach. If it's a heart, breathing, or head problem that persists, seek immediate medical attention. If a physical pain persists beyond a week, schedule an appointment with your doctor.

Feeling Sore?

Depending on your workout experience and activity level, some feel soreness more than others. IF and when you do, the only way for the soreness to subside is for you to do the following three things:

1. Drink .55 times your bodyweight in ounces of water per day. I know this sounds like a lot. Regardless of where you are with it now, just focus on drinking more to work your way closer to this goal. Yes, you will pee a lot at first but your body adapts :).

2. Self-massage: At home, use a rolling pin or a lacrosse, tennis, or softball to roll out the tense areas. It's always good to roll above or below major joints. If you have a sore area, ask us about it and we'll give you more detailed instructions.

3. m.e.l.t.: I know it seems hard to believe when you're sore, but continuing to m.e.l.t. will make you feel better! Your workouts will lubricate your joints and spread your muscle tissue so you will less tension. Plus, you'll feel energized, be more productive throughout the day, and sleep better at night.

How to NEVER Plateau

In your workouts, do a little more each time. This could be more repetitions, a progression of an exercise, more sets—just keep improving.

In your eating habits, eat right 98 percent of the week and enjoy your weekly cheat meal. This will keep your metabolism from slowing.

Always move forward, even when you fall off track. A bad meal or missed workout is not the end of the world; always remember to strive towards gaining momentum, however many times you need to start over.

How to Perform Baseline Movements

Following is a short description of how to perform 4 baseline movements

- Push-Up
- Low Plank
- Hip Hinge
- Squat

Push-Up

Level One

Kneeling Push: Squeeze your upper back muscles, externally rotate your elbows as you drop your chest down to the floor and press up as quickly as you can.

Level Two

Create full body tension as you press your toes into the floor. Squeeze your glutes, squeeze your upper back, externally rotate your elbows as you as you go down partially and push yourself back up.

Level Three

Perform a full range of motion push-up.

Low Plank

Level One — Kneeling

Step 1: Your knees should be slightly behind your hips with your fists directly under your eyeballs and your forearms straight.

Step 2: Achieve ultimate activation by pulling your elbows towards your ribcage.

Step 3: Squeeze your posterior shoulders, your upper back, your glutes.

Step 4: Lock out your legs by squeezing your quads, pressing your toes into the floor, and sucking your bellybutton into your spine, creating a neutral alignment that you must maintain throughout the exercise.

Level Two

Step 1: With your feet touching, extend both legs.

Step 2: Squeeze your glutes to lock your hips and keep them from dropping.

Step 3: Achieve ultimate activation by pulling your elbows towards your ribcage.

Step 4: Squeeze your posterior shoulders, your upper back, and your glutes.

Step 5: Lock out your legs by squeezing your quads, pressing your toes into the floor, and sucking your bellybutton into your spine, creating a neutral alignment that you must maintain throughout the exercise.

Planks should be HARD! Your entire body should be tense, focus on squeezing every part of your body for best results.

Hip Hinge (baseline movement from any deadlift, good morning swing, or high pull)

Pop & Clap

Step 1: With your feet shoulder-width apart, slightly push your knees outward.

Step 2: Sit your butt into your hamstrings (as if someone was pulling your hips back),

Step 3: Simultaneously pop your arms back, maintaining a flat back.

Step 4: Once you feel your hamstrings, push through your heels as you drive your arms forward so your hands are chest level, clap and repeat the first step.

Squat

To practice this movement, use a sturdy and stable object that can support double your body weight to squat onto.

Step 1: Stand with your feet slightly wider than shoulder-width apart.

Step 2: Extend your arms straight out, touching your thumbs together and squeeze your upper back.

Step 3: Sit your butt back into your hamstrings as you push your knees apart.

Step 4: Once you feel your hamstrings, simultaneously bend your knees and squat as low as you can while keeping your upper body tense.

Step 5: Push through your heels and drive your body back up tall.

Do The Best You Can Each Day

Some days you will feel like crushing your workout; other days you will be amazed you dragged yourself to m.e.l.t. On days you feel like you can take on the world, leave it all on the table—there shouldn't be an ounce of energy left in your system. On the days you aren't feeling good, just do what you can.

Remove the pressure of thinking you have to do more.

NEVER doubt yourself - no *"I can't" or "can never."* You can do any movement once you learn the proper form, achieve the stability and strength necessary, and practice.

Feel good about yourself for reading this and committing to m.e.l.t. We will NOT let you fail. Just focus on showing up!

M.E.L.T. PART 3: M.E.L.T. MEAL PLANNING FOR LIFE

Our meal plan is not just a diet where we say, "Hey, eat only XXX and eat like a bird for the rest of your life." No. You work hard and should enjoy life. You can enjoy what you want, 20% of the time, as long as you're following the m.e.l.t. meal plan. We leverage your time so that you're eating clean 80% of the time, and we show you how to do that in a very simple way that's family-friendly. The other 20% of the time you can just do whatever you want as far as eating. The m.e.l.t. Meal Plan allows you to take advantage of doing well and can help you recover from suboptimal choices. You're not going to retract your diet because it's built into your diet.

m.e.l.t. Meal Plan Principals

Diets and most other meal plans end up causing you to gain more belly fat and weight in the long term because they are impossible to sustain. In the m.e.l.t. Meal Plan book, I tell you exactly what to do for any circumstance that comes up. But for the purpose of getting started, we just want to give you the flexibility you need to start achieving balance on all levels. The focus here is to adapt the foundational nutrition principals you need to lose and keep off unwanted weight.

Principal #1 – Schedule Your On Plan/ Off Plan Meals

If you are just getting started on your weight-loss adventure, just focus on following the plan three days on, then taking it easy on the fourth day. That doesn't mean you should binge or completely let go on your fourth day, just don't stress about it as much. You'll repeat this process every four days. Schedule your cheat meals for your fourth day.

If you are regularly exercising, focus on following the plan six days on, one day off. Just like above, the seventh day is not for you to go crazy! Give yourself a little break and enjoy small portions of foods & drinks that you enjoy.

If you're really looking to get to the next level, focus on six days on and one MEAL off. Always give yourself one off meal; it's important to your mind & body that you give yourself some leeway each week.

Give yourself the flexibility to choose the off day. Let's say it's the holidays and a holiday party falls on one of your clean eating days; make that your off day. So if you're doing three days on and one day off and the holiday party falls on a Wednesday, it might look like this:

Mon/Tue	clean eating
Wed	day off
Thur	clean eating
Fri/Sat/Sun	clean eating
Mon	day off

This is just one example. You have the flexibility to make the schedule work for you as long as it's 3 or 6 days of clean eating per week, with only 2 or 1 days off.

Understand there will be times you slip up; just do your best to minimize the damage. When it happens, immediately commit to ONE healthy thing you will do the very next day, such as:

- Drink 18-32 oz. of water
- Prepare a m.e.l.t. meal
- Go for a walk
- Follow the cool down or self-massage routine
- Bonus m.e.l.t. Workout or Yoga

Principal #2 - Pick Your Eating Times

When it comes to developing permanent habits, one of the key components is *ritualizing* the particular habit. You will need to pick an eating frequency that will work for you most of the time. Remember there is no such thing as perfect so if you go down one path and you realize the other frequency might work better, switch.

If you find yourself hungry while following the meal plan, increase the serving size of vegetables. If you are having a hard time following the meal plan, slightly reduce the serving size of each meal. Once you choose a frequency, stick to it – do not skip meals!

Choose the eating frequency option, Option A or Option B, which works best for you.

Option A: 5-6 Smaller Meals (Every Three Hours)

If you are currently only eating once or twice a day, begin by eating 3 or 4 times daily, then move to 5 or 6 times daily; do not go from zero to sixty! Small frequent meals will keep your metabolism and digestion moving so you store fewer calories.

Let's say you wake at 6 a.m. Your eating schedule may look like this:

6:30 a.m.	Breakfast
9:30 a.m.	Morning Snack
12:30 p.m.	Lunch
3:30 p.m.	Afternoon Snack
6:30 p.m.	Dinner
9:30 p.m.	Nighttime Snack*

*The time you eat your last snack depends on when you go to bed. Give your body at least one hour to digest the snack before sleeping. The best nighttime snacks are protein-based, such as Greek yogurt or a hard-boiled egg. Avoid eating grain-based carbohydrates, fruits, and fats after 6 p.m.

Option B: 3 Bigger Meals:

Sometimes frequent eating is not feasible for people who work long hours without breaks. Plan your meals as follows:

Breakfast:	within 1 hour of waking
Lunch:	between 12 to 3 p.m.
Dinner:	between 5 to 7 p.m.

Principal #3 - Hydrate Your Body Sufficiently

Because your body is comprised mostly of water, proper hydration is crucial for you to function at the highest level. Water supports your metabolism, digestion, and elimination;

energizes you, removes toxins, and prevents you from becoming starved.

- How much water should I drink per day?

  Start drinking .55 x your body weight in ounces. Bathroom Cardio is a term I use for going to urinate often when you are properly hydrating. Whether it's 10 feet or 2 floors, walking to the bathroom will awaken your muscles, help your posture, and give your mind a much-needed break, which will boost your productivity. Carry your m.e.l.t. water bottle with you everywhere you go and focus on always filling it up so you drink more water and use less plastic!

- What else can I drink?
  For best results, limit yourself to one coffee and one tea per day. If prefer tea instead of coffee, drink two cups of green or white tea per day. I do recommend you try to limit your coffee consumption to less than 2 cups/day, as too much caffeine can lead to a number of issues, including caffeine over-reliance, sleeping problems, and dehydration. Remember, caffeine is a diuretic and has the net effect of dehydrating you!

- What can I add to my coffee or tea?
  Only add cinnamon, coconut or nut milk, stevia, or 1 teaspoon of honey to your hot drink.

Stop drinking your calories! Remove these liquids from your diet:

- **Juices or juice-flavored drinks**. This includes chemically altered sugar-free drinks such as Crystal Light.

- **Diet branded shakes** (for example, Slim-fast).

- **All sodas, including diet**. Even diet soda will raise your insulin levels, cause you to become hungry, and lead to fat gain.

- **Sports drinks**. Sports drinks are designed to be consumed only after excessive sweating. And remember that a typical sports drink bottle usually has several servings in it.

- **Alcohol**. If you booze, you will not lose (pounds)! For best results, limit alcohol consumption to 1 or 2 alcoholic drinks a week. But know that even just 1 or 2 drinks a week will prevent you from having the flat stomach you desire. For some people 1-2 drinks per week is much harder than others; it's not all or nothing, if you're having a nightly cocktail, first reduce it to every other day, then every second day.

Principal #4 - Eliminate Processed and Garbage Foods

Eat only whole foods or foods closest to their origin. You will find most of these foods along the perimeter of the grocery store in the produce, dairy and meats / poultry / fish sections.

Avoid Fast Food:

Even the 200-calorie items can cause damage because they're loaded with unnatural components which slow down your metabolism & digestion.

Clear Your Kitchen of Food Traps:

- Protein bars (also known as glorified candy bars) or "nutritional" bars with more than 10 ingredients and 10 grams of sugar

- Foods with hydrogenated oil or high-fructose corn syrup in the ingredients – check all crackers, cereals, fries, oils, spreads, dressings and sauces - even 100 calorie packs and "gluten free" varieties

- Desserts (even reduced sugar or sugar-free desserts). Although we recommend you enjoy things you love, have them in proportion and only once a week. But if you have it lying around your house, you will eat it! In addition, reduced-sugar desserts are created from artificial sweeteners that trick your brain and trigger hunger.

- Refined Vegetable oils (canola, corn, soybean, sunflower, safflower, Crisco)

Make Healthier Choices:

- Start shopping around the perimeter of the grocery store. Buy fresh and frozen whole foods to cook on your own.

- Obtain flavor from healthful sources!

    - Cinnamon
    - Spices
    - Hot peppers
    - Low Sodium Hot Sauce
    - Lemon zest
    - Fresh fruits or veggies (guacamole, salsa, and so on.)

- Extra Virgin Olive Oil
- Red Wine Vinaigrette or Apple Cider Vinegar

So get ready to jump-start your nutrition with those four principals! For an exact blueprint of everything you need from an eating plan, check out our m.e.l.t. Meal Plan Book. With that book, you get:

- What to eat
- How to eat for best results
- What you need to know about supplements
- Tips to increase your metabolism
- Tips for staying on track when eating out at restaurants
- Tips for eating on the go
- Tasty – healthily – fast recipes
- Strategies for working the m.e.l.t. meal plan into your life
- List of "free foods"

M.E.L.T. PART 4: THE M.E.L.T. LIFESTYLE

The m.e.l.t. lifestyle is not about telling you to live a certain way. It's about showing you the shortest path towards the body you seek and incorporating a growth mindset, results-maximizing workouts, and healthy eating habits into your life style.

Where Everybody Knows Your Name

The second you join m.e.l.t., you become part of an extended family. Our #meltfamily is something bigger than yourself– it's a group of like-minded people where together we can accomplish more than we could ever dream of as individuals.

Whether it's participating in our charitable efforts, getting and giving daily support from fellow members, or just the friendly atmosphere that allows you to put down your guard so you can open up for growth, you'll feel like a part of our community.

New hires and new m.e.l.t.ers are always amazed by how friendly everyone is. The reason everyone is so friendly is that everyone wants to be here—because m.e.l.t. is more than just a gym.

You never have to worry about doing your hair and makeup, or wearing designer gear for a workout. No one here will judge you—just show up as you are.

A big mistake people make is they think they have to get in

shape just to be able to work out. That's the worst and the most wrong thing you could ever think. Our Rock Star Michelle got in shape by coming to m.e.l.t. In only seven months, she's lost over 120 pounds and she's the talk and pride of m.e.l.t. And that's because she lost all the weight and because fellow m.e.l.t.ers see her give her best at every workout.

Michelle appeared on TV with m.e.l.t., on a Better Connecticut segment, and had the courage to share her journey with tens of thousands of viewers! Seven months ago she would have felt too self-conscious, but today she's on TV talking about her success. I think Michelle's story shows that you can achieve anything. You've just got to take that first step forward.

You Are Never Alone

The family-like atmosphere has created some AMAZING bonds over the years. We've had m.e.l.t.ers become best friends, we've even had two people meet at m.e.l.t. and get engaged. While marriages aren't common, the vibe is that regardless of whether you're looking for friendship or you just want to work out—you are never alone.

> *"You are the average of the five people you spend the most time with."*
>
> \- *Jim Rohn*

Just recently a m.e.l.t.er's husband was diagnosed with a serious form of cancer. Without hesitation, several m.e.l.t.ers set up a bank account to raise funds for their family and a created a meal service to help cook for their children. It was amazing to see m.e.l.t.ers who didn't even know the family go out of their way to help.

Connecting With Your #meltfamily Facebook Page

The #meltfamily Facebook page is THE place to connect with your fellow m.e.l.t.ers. Every day you'll find something positive:

- **Share progress**: Acknowledging progress will lead to more progress. The outside world confuses this with bragging. Inside m.e.l.t., we encourage you to share your progress because it motivates and inspires others.
- **Post questions**: Whether it's about nutrition, events, or training questions—there's always someone knowledgeable to help
- **Share recipes**: Our m.e.l.t.ers are happy to pass along delicious, on-plan, family-friendly recipes.
- **Share vulnerability**: We've had people share the struggles they've gone or are going through, which you just don't share unless you feel trust. But when you do share, you feel like a weight has been lifted off you and you open yourself up for growth.
- **Make each other laugh**: There always seems to be a funny meme about working out or a video. Just recently we had a m.e.l.t.er do a spoof video of working out as Godzilla at home on a snow day for no other reason than to make others laugh. And it was hilarious.
- **Find running buddies**: You'll find m.e.l.t.ers at just about every local adventure race and 5K who are open to register together as a m.e.l.t. team, train with each other, carpool, and hold each other accountable.

Just about any type of event you'd want to do, you can find someone within the m.e.l.t. family to do it with!

Work Hard, Train Hard, Play Hard

We believe that you need to enjoy the fruits of your labor—whatever that means to you. It's sad to see people become so obsessed with fitness that they are scared to do anything to damage their progress. The good news is it doesn't have to be like that. With the m.e.l.t. Workout, down time/recovery is built into our program, as is cheating or indulging in the things you love.

#melt IT Forward

Watch the news for three minutes and you will be convinced we live in a screwed-up world with screwed-up people. I don't like the news for this very reason—the news is televised not to inform but to scare. The media want you to think things are bad just so you keep tuning in. While the world is not perfect, the reality is there are a lot of good people in this world doing good things.

Once your oxygen mask is on, you can use your strength to help others, and there is no better feeling in this world. And at m.e.l.t. we are all about feeling good.

#m.e.l.t.ITForward is our volunteering and fundraising effort centered around giving back and paying it forward. It's our ongoing campaign where m.e.l.t.ers are welcome to join in all types of events ranging from hosting charity workouts, handing out roses to the elderly, volunteering in the community, collecting toys/food—you name it. It's easy to think when you're one person that your contribution will not make an impact; however, the collective effort of a group like the #meltfamily can do some pretty amazing things.

When your fitness becomes something more than just exercising, it becomes part of your life and the narrative around exercise changes. It's no longer "if you work out," it's "when you work out"—which is why most m.e.l.t.ers get into the best shape of their lives.

What Else do You Want to Accomplish?

Yes, at the core we are a fitness facility—but we're also here to help you transform your life. Once you start feeling good, you're going ignite something inside you didn't know existed. We encourage you to use this new-found energy in all other aspects of your life.

Here's a list of activities we'd like to see our m.e.l.t.ers make part of their lifestyle:

1. Travel more: Doesn't have to be exotic, there are plenty of places to see in New England!
2. Spend more time with family
3. Make fitness a family effort. Remember it's about a lifestyle! We love seeing family members join or come to charity workouts. We want you to send in pictures of you and your family m.e.l.t.ing at home or on vacation.
4. Learn how to cook
5. Experiment with new foods
6. Cook more often
7. Incorporate yoga into your routine
8. Hike
9. Bike

10. Play recreational sports
11. Read more
12. Volunteer
13. Advance your career

These are just the more common activities we suggest – what is it that *you* want to do? A part of m.e.l.t.ing is realizing how much you are capable of and getting out there and doing it. We can't wait to help you succeed!

Fear and procrastination are the enemies of success.

CASE STUDIES

Melt30™

At Home Fat loss & Strength DVD

Leeann K

I dropped 10 pounds and 14.25 total inches in JUST 8 weeks!

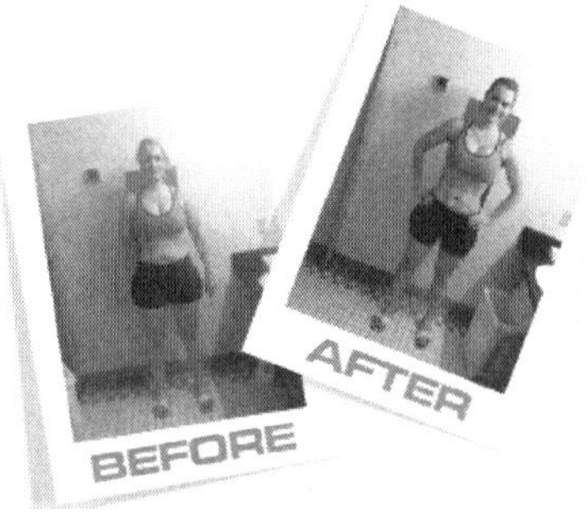

I feel AMAZING! my confidence is coming back. It feels great to buy new clothes that are "sexy" instead of buying clothes to hide my body. I am more positive. I try to help co-workers and friends with their struggle with weight loss, I am happier and am much more energetic.

And for the first time since high school I LOVE working out again.

Before m.e.l.t., I didn't want to do anything; had low energy; was overweight; had trouble sleeping and no confidence.

I tried big gyms with machines; long bootcamp type classes that was all cardio work; other workout videos such as Julian Michaels and Hip hop abs and nothing worked.

I had an unexpected medical procedure any my recovery

period took longer than expected, I ended up gaining more weight and felt discouraged.

When i saw an ad for MELT and it was only 30 minutes so thought it was worth a shot.

I have gained strength and endurance; am no longer tired all the time and am sleeping better. (Although I didn't see weight loss right away) I did notice my body toning. In just 8 weeks with MELT, I dropped 10 pounds and 14.25 total inches.

MELT is the way to go! Big box gyms and a lot of other dvds are cookie cutter. M.e.l.t. concentrates on all body parts and gives you variations of the exercises so it's great for all fitness levels. You have nothing to lose (but weight) by trying it out..

Friends, Family and co-workers can't believe the change. I haven't seen my grandmother in a few months and when I saw her she actually said to "your melting away". Love that everyone around me notices the big change; that attention is something that I've missed.

The best part of that is it is bringing my confidence level back. I'm not hiding in a shell anymore.

MELT is the way to go! Big box gyms and a lot of other dvds are cookie cutter. M.e.l.t. concentrates on all body parts gives you variations of the exercises so it's great for all fitness levels. You have nothing to lose (but weight) by trying it out.

I always look forward to my m.e.l.t. Workouts. The Motivation, energy and drive is something I look forward to at the end of a long stressful day at work.

I work "a lot" pretty much from time I wake up to time I go to bed. But with the 30 minute workouts it gives me that small break from the "work world" and re-energizes me. Other programs and workout DVD's are too long (longer than 30 minutes); not motivational and become boring after doing them for a week. MELT always gives you something different so it doesn't get old.

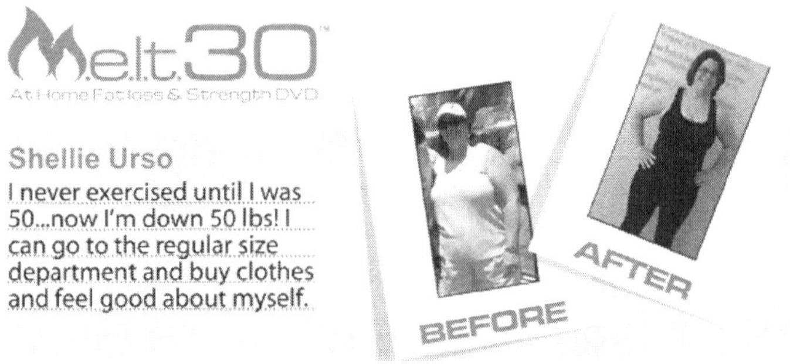

My sister, Kelley, told me I had to try the m.e.l.t. Workout....she said it was "The Workout" if I was looking to get "hooked" into a program and actually see results.

Before I started m.e.l.t.. I was seeing minimal results with a personal trainer at LA Fitness then my sessions ended I knew I couldn't do it on my own.

My sister, Kelley, told me I had to try the m.e.l.t. Workout....she said it was "The Workout" if I was looking to get "hooked" into a program and actually see results.

I have lost a total of 50 pounds and now trying to keep myself in shape and lose 20 pounds more which will be the lowest I have been since I had my children 25 years ago. I look forward to my workouts and miss them when I'm on vacation.

I feel pretty fantastic, especially since before I started the m.e.l.t. Workout I didn't want to exercise at all. I have learned a lot about myself and what I can accomplish in my 50's and know that I can still keep up with my daughters and younger sister.

I feel that I have the energy to do anything. It is very important to me to keep exercising for my health and well-being and be able to someday be around

for my grandchildren. I want to be able to stay as active as possible well into my 80's. Now I want to be more conscious of my diet to match my workout and not be ashamed of my look.

I never exercised before I was 50. I hated to even walk for exercise so I let myself go and gained a ton of weight and started having health issues. I also never went on diets. I just ate what I wanted to and didn't care so getting the education that you provide and the workout routines have saved my life.

My older daughter bugged me for years to exercise and lose weight and she is so happy now that I take care of myself and because she's such a workout and diet girl, we now have something in common about workouts and how we eat. I'm so happy when friends or even people that don't know me tell me how great I look. I'm so humbled by that I don't know what to say except thanks.

There's no better feeling then making my daughters proud. Personally it feels amazing that I can go to the regular size department and buy clothes and feel good about myself.

Not only is m.e.l.t. do able, it is only 30 minutes and has a high energy exercises that keep you motivated to keep going and your food plan is not just a diet but a new beginning to eat right and stay on course for losing weight and maintaining weight. Joe's enthusiasm is contagious and that you want to workout with him. He really cares about you and wants you to be the best person you can become.

The workouts are challenging and keep my interest because there is always something new everyday and the workouts attack every body part. I want the workouts to be harder and I want my body to be better....I never would have felt like this before m.e.l.t.ing.

Because my work life is so incredibly intense, I need to take a break and "MELT". I feel that I am getting personal training and I am releasing the stress and breakaway that I need before I go to work.

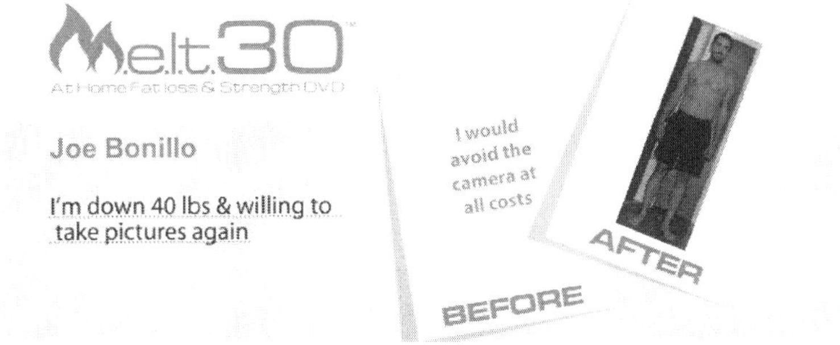

I still use both sets of pictures as motivation and I WISH I had taken those 20lb heavier before pictures. Regardless, I see tremendous development even in those last 25 lbs

When I was 220lbs I didn't take any before pictures despite their advice to do so. In fact, I didn't really want to be in any pictures so I haven't been able to really find one that shows where I was. I didn't take the pictures for a couple reasons. 1) I didn't want pictures of me at that weight. It was not pretty. 2) I hadn't stuck with a workout plan EVER and so I wasn't confident that there would need to be AFTER pictures. 3) I was simply embarrassed by my body and lacked the confidence to stand in front of a camera with my shirt off.

After losing 20 lbs and feeling more confident I took "before" pictures so I could see the results going forward. I have lost 25lbs since then and have worked to target certain areas even after my "after" pictures but they are a fair representation of where I'm at.

I know they aren't as drastic as some work out promotions you see on TV where the person now has a 6-pack. I think the difference in my case is that there was so much neglect for three decades that it is going to take more than one year of healthy eating/living to remove it all. So when you use these pictures I would like that to be the message...if you are out of shape like I was it simply takes hard work, dedication to the program, and time. Not awesome selling points for a society that loves easy fixes. But I will say this...the MELT program gave me better, faster results than anything I had even done before.

I still use both sets of pictures as motivation and I WISH I had taken those 20lb heavier before pictures. Regardless, I see tremendous development even in those last 25 lbs.

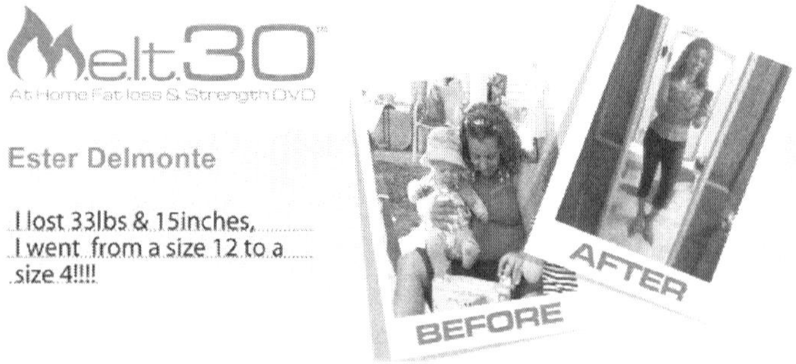

I am now where I always wanted to be! I am happy and my body feels great and I love my new me!!!! I have more energy I'm excited for each day, I sleep better and I feel like life is much easier now!

Before I started the m.e.l.t. program, I was at my ONE year mark after having my baby and my body felt like I was still 6 months pregnant.

I tried taking the baby out for walking, I tried 3 different diets and, I also rode my bike, but nothing seemed to work. Then I saw all the progress one of my best friends was making so I asked her what she was doing and she said "m.e.l.ting!"

I am now where I always wanted to be! I am happy and my body feels great and I love my new me!!!! I have more energy I'm excited for each day, I sleep better and I feel like life is much easier now!

It feels good getting compliments from the people I love, and they saw my struggles when I couldn't get out of my rut!

The workout is unlike any other; short, high energy and the coaches enthusiasms!!! The 30 minute m.e.l.tWorkouts are easy for me to fit into my busy schedule and I look forward to each of them!

m.e.l.t.30
At Home Fat loss & Strength DVD

Jeff Hill

Far Leaner Now With These 30 Minute m.e.l.t. Workouts Than The Hours I Use To Spend At The Local Gym.

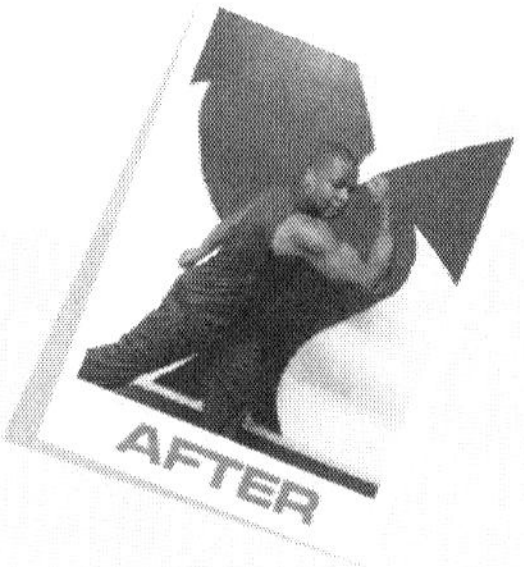

My turning point was finding out about the m.e.l.t. Workout, what intially attracted me were realizing a lot of what I was doing physically and what I was eating, were wrong. I am now maximizing my workout in less time. I have more energy and all my old strains/ injuries have never felt better! As a former athlete, I am proud to say I am in the best shape of my life, far leaner now in these 30 minute workouts then the hours I use to spend at the local gym.

I use to go to the gym regularly, spending 1-2 hours. I would do the same routine/exercise all the time and from time to time I would often sustain injuries due to improper form and techniques. I had the right mindset but the wrong approach. Before m.e.l.t.

I thought I was eating healthy yet my sodium levels were through the roof...as it turns out, I wasn't eating as healthy was I thought I was.

My turning point was finding out about the m.e.l.t. Workout, what intially attracted me were realizing a lot of what I was doing physically and what I was eating, were wrong. I am now maximizing my workout in less time. I have more energy and all my old strains/ injuries have never felt better!

As a former athlete, I am proud to say I am in the best shape of my life, far leaner now in these 30 minute workouts then the hours I use to spend at the local gym.

I feel great! I have been amazed by what I have been able to accomplish in less time.

My life has definitely changed for the better. I feel less stress. My mood is more upbeat. My primary care doctor has been amazed at the results of my annual physical exams....I am no longer taking blood pressure meds!

People in my life often comment about how fit I look. My ability to lead and inspire others at work has greatly improved, a direct result of the m.e.l.t. Workouts.

I have more endurance. I can lift more weights than I could before. I have also experienced more physical flexibility than I have in the past....this has dramatically helped the shoulder and low back pain I use to chronically suffer from.

When I first started m.e.l.t.ing, family n friends use to comment all the time about my transformation...now I think they are just use to seeing my fit and healthy! But I still get comments from random people I run into, like grocery shopping, who are amazed at my physique.

Melt has been very instrumental in helping me health and fitness a priority in my life.

If you are looking to see fast results, you need to give the M.E.L.T. workout a try, your search will be over.... you will get everything you need to help you accomplish your fitness goals with their DVD and online training resources.

Melt workouts are definitely fun and keep my interest. The coach is passionate and keeps it fun. ...you feel comfortable regardless of your fitness level. The workouts are innovative and engaging so you are always motivated to work hard and to maximize your fitness goals.

The passion, care and concern of MELT keeps me engaged.

The 30 minute m.e.l.t.Workouts leaves more time for you to devote to other things in your life that are equally as important; more time to spend with family, friends and doing other things that you enjoy doing.

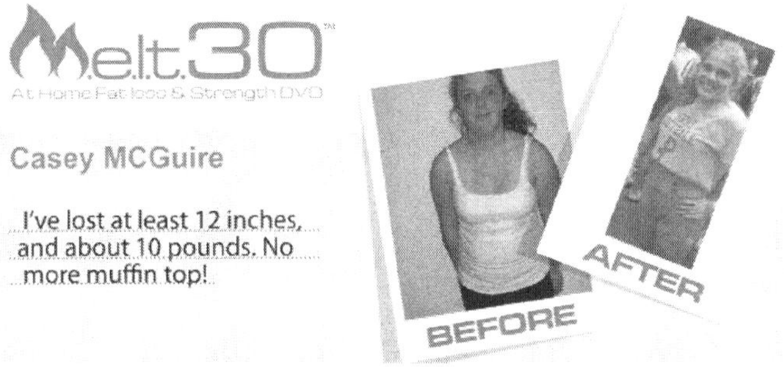

I started m.e.l.t.ing because of my mom...she loved the workouts, and they were making a difference for her. I saw her change, and her attitude, and after much urging from her, tried it for myself. After my first workout, I was hooked.

Before m.e.l.t.ing, I was the average high school student – playing one sport, dancing, and skiing, with the ability to participate in all, but nothing special, and not in what I would call "good shape." And without really realizing it, I'd begun to sprout a "muffin top."

The workouts really make me work up a sweat, and challenge me to work hard. M..e.l.t. makes it feel like we're all together, like I'm a part of the group on the screen, getting encouragement from the coach.

As a high school student, I was busy, and getting the average amount of exercise, but it clearly wasn't enough.

I started m.e.l.t.ing because of my mom...she loved the workouts, and they were making a difference for her. I saw her change, and her attitude, and after much urging from her, tried it for myself. After my first workout, I was hooked!

I've lost at least 12 inches, and about 10 pounds. No more muffin top! I love my new body and I've totally changed my eating habits to maintain my new self. I work out at least 6x/week and friends say I'm "ripped." For the first time ever this year, I challenged myself to do some 5k's (one at a time-never thought I'd do more than 1) and even 3 fitness 5k's! This has changed my life.

I love the way my clothes fit and the way I look in pictures.

I never entered races before. Now I look for more! I did my first one reluctantly, from peer pressure and walked for most of it. But after that, I've never had to walk, and I love it! I did my first couple with family, but my latest 2 I found friends to do it with me, and left my family home! I'm much more confident in general.

A lot of family and friends comment on how great I look, and how I've adopted better eating habits. They also say I'm an inspiration to them. My new confidence has strangers in the gym commenting about how positive I am, and how I inspire them.

I love the attention I get from family and friends, commenting on how fit I look. And I love that others find me inspirational. I hope others can do MELT and feel as good about themselves as I feel about my transformation.

You won't regret getting this DVD. It's awesome and you will definitely see results if you stick to it. It's not hard to stick to, and it's fun to do! You need to be in it to win it!

m.e.l.t.30™
At Home Fat loss & Strength DVD

Brooke Trombley
I had tried it all and nothing worked until m.e.l.t.: I'm down 54lbs and 3, almost 4, pant sizes!!!

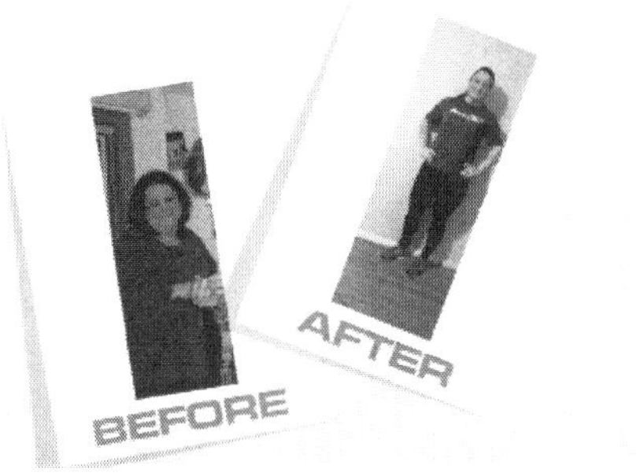

I have more energy and attempt things I never thought I would do. I am getting ready to run my first 5k in the spring. I do things in m.e.l.t. I never thought I could do. I love it!

I was always tired full of excuses, never wanting to go anywhere or do anything. It was always "I,ll start tomorrow." I was considered obese and embarrassed about it.

I tried several different diets may have lost 5lbs or so but within no time the weight was back. I did weight watchers,diet pills, gym memberships, Wii, other videos that took forever and were so boring! Nothing worked for me or at least keep my interest long enough to keep sticking with them.

My "just go for it" moment was when I got a text message from my girlfriend that had been m.e.l.t.ing for a few months asking me if I wanted to m.e.l.t. that night with her. Ill admit I was put on the spot but have never been happier to have gotten that message and replying YES!! Haven't looked back since.

I have been m.e.l.t.ing for 6 months and I'm down 54lbs

and 3, almost 4, pant sizes. I have more energy and attempt things I never thought I would do. I am getting ready to run my first 5k in the spring. I do things in m.e.l.t. I never thought I could do. I love it!

It makes me feel amazing...able to hold my head up high. It's made me a better mother to my 3 children getting me more involved with them. Able to jump on the bike and take a ride around the block with out them having to stop and wait for me, playing in the back yard with out complaining that I was out of breath or my legs hurt. Its a whole new life!

I'm doing burppies, planks,speed squats, kettle bells, I could go on and on. I never thought I could do any of the things I do while m.e.l.t.ing. I never had the confidence to even try. I have confidence now! M.e.l.t.ing has changed my life in so many ways. I'm happy!!

My friends and family have been great! It definitely doesn't get old hearing all the compliments.

It makes me feel alive finally that I'm not just a body I'm a person. It just boost that confidence even more. Confidence I never had.

I would say what are you waiting for??? M.e.l.t. has different levels for all types of people. There is nothing to lose but weight. Its a 1/2 hr of work and a lifetime of happiness! Start slow and work your way up challenge yourself. You will be amazed at the results.

The work outs are great! I don't think I could pin point 1 specific part that keeps me engaged, I enjoy everything. I like to try and challenge myself, and

the motivation that you get ables you to challenge yourself and you can do it!

I am a mother of 3 and work fulltime. My oldest son who is 13 plays travel hockey we are at the arena 4 days a week traveling at least 1 of those days to the other end of that state. My other son is 7 and my daughter is 1. Time was not a part of my vocabulary. That was always my excuse "I don't have time!!" Guess what I have time, its a 1/2hr. I didn't have 2-3hrs to go to the gym I still don't but doing a 30min M.e.l.t gives me more results anyhow then spending hours on end at the gym. There are no more excuses, set your alarm a 1/2hr early, don't sit on the couch and watch that 1/2 hr of T.V. Involve your family do it together. You can always find a 1/2hr to work out to feel great for the other 23 1/2hours of the day. Once you start your not going to want to stop, it just becomes part of you. You look forward to that 1/2hr!

Melt30™
At Home Fat loss & Strength DVD

Beth C.

I I've lost 22 pounds and have maintained my new weight!

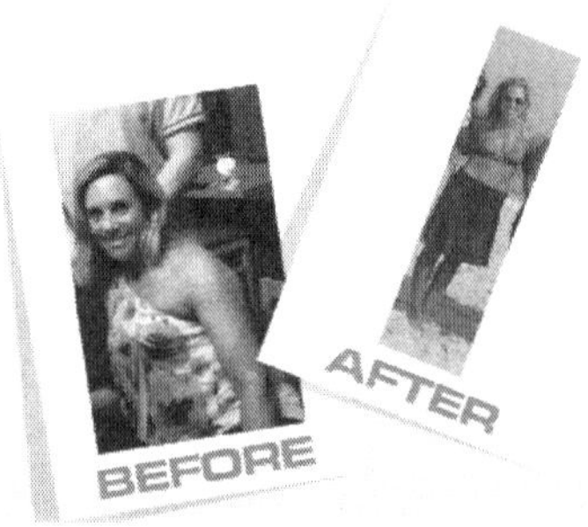

I am stronger and more toned than I have been since I was a teenager and most importantly I release any stress I have during my workouts, which makes me feel better and make better food choices later.

Before I started m.e.l.t.ing I was in a funk. I was going through a divorce, and unlike most people who lose weight when they are stressed, I gained! The holidays killed me, and I continued eating after them. I couldn't button most of the pants in my closet, and the ones I could button, I thought made me look huge and out of shape. One day I realized I WAS larger than what I had been used to, and I WAS out of shape!

Before m.e.l.t. my workout routine was very inconsistent. I ran, but only in the nice weather, I used my elliptical in the basement, but only when nothing else in my house was more interesting, and I did Shred (Jillian Michaels), which would have been good if the most challenging level she had was her beginner level. I got bored.

The moment I realized I needed to take control of my out of control body was when I noticed the only place I had never struggled with weight gain in the past had grown inches - my waist. My friend and I were both down about how we felt and happened to come across an advertisement for what seemed to be a motivating workout, m.e.l.t. It was going to take a lot to motivate me, but we decided it was worth a try. I needed to fit in my clothes again!

I have been m.e.l.t.ing now for exactly one year! I lost 22 pounds and have maintained my new weight, which is the biggest challenge! In two months I lost 2.5 inches in my waist and hips! I am stronger and more toned than I have been since I was a teenager and most importantly I release any stress I have during my workouts, which makes me feel better and make better food choices later.

I have changed physically in many ways -- I'm stronger, I have defined muscles in places I didn't think women could have muscles, I challenge myself independently and I WANT to workout.

I crave the workouts, and when I can't get them in because of life "getting in the way" I don't feel 100%. m.e.l.t. helped me through something I couldn't have done on my own. I got through my divorce, a very difficult time in my life, by taking care of myself in mind and body, through my daily workouts. It's amazing what punching a bag, tire flipping and medicine ball slams can do for your mental and emotional health, as well as your physical health!

My friends and family are amazed at the transformation I have made, and when asked how I lost the weight and got such defined shoulders and arms, I tell them I m.e.l.t!

The best part about this for me is that I have a sense of

confidence I have never had before, and I am learning to accept the compliments because it IS true. I feel like a million bucks! M.e.l.t's program and dedication to clients' weight loss and transformation process paired with my hard work has changed me, and it's something to be proud of and share!

I have been doing m.e.l.t. workouts for one year, and have never gotten bored, or thought "time to switch to a different program." Each workout is unique, to focus on specific areas of the body.

Everyone's life is busy, so fitting in a full body workout into 30 minutes is ideal and was one of the biggest selling points for me. Having three children involved in multiple activities themselves in not conducive to long workouts. The best part is, 30 minutes is all you need with the m.e.l.t. workout!

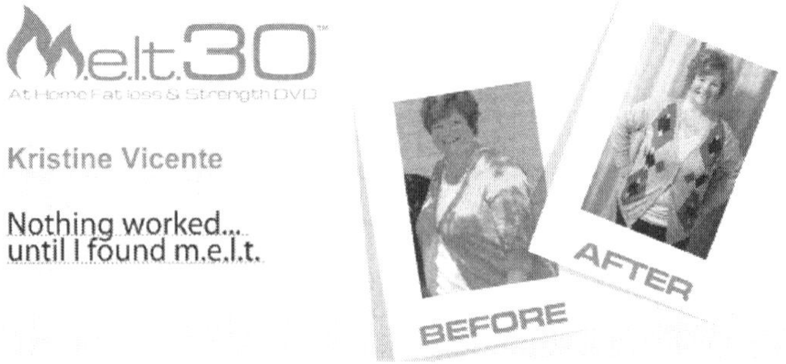

> My family, my friends, my co-workers see that my clothes are too big and notice the new glow to my skin and ask me if I've been working out. I'm so proud to say "yes!"

I've been very overweight for 15+ years and sitting at a desk job for 40+ hours a week hasn't helped. I was sore, achy, weak and lethargic. It was hard to get motivated but I knew I had to do something to get the weight off and to start moving more because my health was in jeopardy.

Before M.E.L.T. I tried walking, running, yoga, Curves, big box gyms and many different diet plans. Everything I tried took up too much time and/or wasn't very effective. I don't really enjoy exercising so I wasn't really pushing myself to do more, until I found M.E.L.T.

I heard about m.e.l.t. from one of my best friends who transformed her life through the program. I felt like the workout was so intense and extremely efficient for the amount of time it took up that I would make the commitment to myself to put in the 30 minutes 4x a week to get on a path to a healthier me. I decided that even if the movement was a struggle for me, I would work the modification until I could do the full movement and always do my best every session.

Right now I've been doing M.E.L.T. 4x per week for about 6 months. I've lost about 15 pounds and a total of 7 inches–3 inches off my waist and 4 inches off my hips.I feel like it's really paying off, I feel better today than I have in years! I marvel at the amount of energy I have and the muscle tone that's becoming more obvious to me and to others.

I feel so happy and so grateful. I feel like this program has given me the kind of workout push I need to stay motivated. I love that people are noticing my weight loss and the toning of my body despite the fact that I have at least 60 pounds to go! I know I can do it with this program. The variety of movements keeps me interested and engaged. I never get bored.

I'm already I'm noticing small things, like the energy I still have after cleaning the house, being able to run up the two flights of stairs to my office without getting winded, the loose waist on my pants. I LOVE that! I feel more confident and I feel more self-caring because I know that every time I M.E.L.T. I'm doing something good for myself, something to keep me strong and healthy.

My family, my friends, my co-workers see that my clothes are too big and notice the new glow to my skin and ask me if I've been working out. I'm so proud to say "yes!".

It feels good to know that I have found a way to exercise that challenges me and pushes me to do my best every time.

You can't get a better workout in 30 minutes then with the m.e.l.t. program.

The workotus absolutely fun and keep me interested. I feel like every part of the session is engaging–the warm-up gets my muscle groups activated, the exercises themselves keep me challenged, focused and doing my best to keep good form and execute them properly for both safety and effectiveness...my favorite part is the stretch at the end because my muscles are warm and tingling and I know I just did something great for my body! I love the improvement I've seen in my execution of the exercises over the last 6 months. They show me I really am getting stronger and more fit!

The intensity of the M.E.L.T. 30 minute workouts give you a lot of exercise in a short amount of time. I make a point of fitting in my workouts early in my day before anything can get in the way of that time. I really look forward to the workouts because I know every time I workout I'm a little bit closer to reaching my fitness goals. I'm already seeing the results of this effort.

Maria Zarrilo

I have lost 21 pounds in 6 weeks, I am down 2 sizes in my clothes, my knees and feet don't hurt anymore, I have so much energy and I notice that the exercises that were a little more difficult when I first started to m.e.l.t. are getting easier. While I still have ways to go, with m.e.l.t. I now know I can get there.

It makes me feel amazing. I catch myself looking in the mirror quite often because I never believed I could look or feel this different. It feels wonderful knowing that i am healthier than I was yesterday!!!

I was really heading down a road of destruction, i could hardly walk sometimes my knees hurt so bad, i was tired all the time; I figured I was too over weight to ever be able to physically be able to do what was needed to be able to lose weight, with the 30 minute workouts 3 times a week, i have lost 21 pounds in 6 weeks (even though the holidays) and feel so amazing, it is hard to put into words.

Before trying m.e.l.t. I tried going to the gym, doing the elliptical or walking on the treadmill but i never really found the inner ambition to keep going, I just would get bored and find every reason not to go. I honestly look forward to m.e.l.ting, there are so many different exercises you can do, and it makes it more interesting and fun.

I have a friend who lost a considerable amount of weight and was looking really good. She told me with her busy schedule she did a 30 minute workout 4 days a week and suggested I try it. I figured if it worked for her it could work for me as we generally were often as busy as the other. M.e.l.t. has worked for her and it is for me.

I have lost 21 pounds in 6 weeks, i am down 2 sizes in my clothes, my knees and feet don't hurt anymore, i have so much more energy and i notice that the exercises that were a little more difficult when i first started to m.e.l.t. are getting easier.

It makes me feel amazing. I catch myself looking in the mirror quite often because I never believed I could look or feel this different. It feels wonderful knowing that i am healthier than I was yesterday!!!

The new me has changed my life!!! I feel like a total different person, i can walk up the stairs now without feeling like I am going to die, I can get on the floor and play with my dog and not worry about "how am I going to get up off the floor". I am more confident in myself; i know that if i can overcome my weight issue, i can overcome just about anything because "i can do anything i put my mind to".

My family and friends are always saying things to me that make me feel so good that I want to continue to do more, for me; because those things are nice to hear.

My family and friends told me that they were really

starting to worry about me and my overall health.

The best part about family and friends complementing on the new me makes me realize what good i am doing for myself.

If you even got to the point to inquire about a home weight loss / energy solution you are ready!!! Do it for yourself, you are so worth it. Little changes make big results and the program is friendly for beginners and non-beginners.

I really sincerely love the m.e.l.t. workouts, there are so many different exercises to do that it never gets redundant or boring, if you are having an off day you can do a less intense workout and if you are feeling energized and pumped you can do an exercise that is a little bit more challenging.

The m.e.l.t workouts are only 30 minutes, I tell myself all the time "you are worth 30 minutes" and the fact that I really enjoy them makes me not even think twice about not making the time to go. I would make excuses all the time before I discovered m.e.l.t. not to workout, now especially after seeing amazing results, I know I can do this because I've already have proven to myself with my results so far and with my busy lifestyle I will continue to m.e.l.t.

RESOURCES FOR YOU

1. **M30 Greens**

- 12 servings of fruits and veggies in ONE scoop!
- Easily mix your greens and water in seconds - the quickest and healthiest on-the-go snack for busy days.
- It tastes more like a fruit drink with the benefits of vegetables and zero empty calories (these add unnecessary amounts of extra fat).
- Hit 2 birds with 1 stone by adding it to your protein shake for a filling and balanced meal replacement.
- Improve absorption and digestion with the proprietary probiotic complex and digestive enzyme blend.
- You'll rarely get sick!!! These specialized greens strengthen your immune system with the antioxidants, herbs & detoxifiers to prevent nasty viruses from ruining your week.
- Enjoy on the go - GUILT FREE!

Order yours at www.meltgreens.com

2. **m.e.l.t. At Home Fat Loss & Strength Workout System**

- 9 Workouts that target your trouble areas allowing you to get toned up in minutes a day:
    - Belly Fat m.e.l.t.er
    - Fat Attack Bootcamp

  - Fat m.e.l.t.ing Bootcamp
  - Stomach Shredder
  - Upper Body Sculptor
  - Lower Body Sculptor
  - Push Series for Triceps, Legs, Chest & Shoulders
  - Pull Series for Biceps, Butt & Back
  - The Zen m.e.l.t.er
- Fitness Guide
- Video Vault of Exercise Demonstrations

Order the digital and/or physical copy at www.meltathome.com

3. **Book Joe to speak at your next event!**

Joe will show your people how to:

- Develop a positive mindset to accomplish more
- How to get more energy in less time
- How to Workout anywhere and achieve results no matter how busy you are
- To be more productive and less stress
- Increases their self-confidence and feel accomplished

To get more information, email info@meltfitnessstudio.com

19579989R00062

Made in the USA
Middletown, DE
26 April 2015